# Contents

# 1 Introduction to Neuro-Ophthalmology

Neuro-ophthalmology sits at the fascinating intersection of neurology and ophthalmology, a crucial area impacting patients' vision and overall well-being. It's a field where understanding the intricate neural pathways responsible for sight is paramount to effective diagnosis and treatment. The intricate dance between the brain and the eye, often overlooked in individual specialty practices, forms the very basis of this multifaceted discipline.

Consider the visual pathway itself—a complex series of interconnected structures that transmit visual information from the retina to the brain. Damage at any point in this pathway can lead to a range of visual disturbances, emphasizing the need for a comprehensive understanding of both neurological and ophthalmological principles. This interdisciplinary approach demands collaborative efforts, merging the skills of neurologists, ophthalmologists, and other specialists to deliver holistic patient care.

Historically, neuro-ophthalmology emerged from a need to clarify the connection between neurological dysfunction and visual impairments. Early observations of patients with neurological diseases exhibiting vision problems paved the way for this dedicated field. Pioneering work gradually unraveled the complex relationships, revealing the intricate link between visual perception and brain function. Further advancements in imaging technology and our growing understanding of neuroanatomy have dramatically enhanced our ability to diagnose and manage a wide array of neuro-ophthalmological conditions.

The meticulous examination of the visual pathway, from the light-sensitive cells of the retina to the visual cortex, forms the cornerstone of any assessment. Detailed knowledge of the optic nerve, optic chiasm, optic tracts, lateral geniculate nucleus, and optic radiations is essential for accurately interpreting the specific location and nature of any lesion affecting the visual system. Such expertise requires a thorough grasp of anatomical structures and their functional significance, allowing clinicians to pinpoint the exact point of disruption within the pathway.

Clinical practice in neuro-ophthalmology involves a careful combination of history taking, thorough ophthalmologic examination, and neurological assessment. The detailed history should explore the nature, onset, and progression of visual symptoms; identifying any other associated neurological deficits that might suggest a broader systemic issue. Ophthalmological examination requires precise assessment of visual acuity, visual fields, pupillary responses, and extraocular movements, identifying any subtle abnormalities that might escape less-focused examinations. Neurological examination provides additional insights, helping determine the possible location and extent of neurological involvement.

Advanced imaging techniques significantly enhance the diagnostic capabilities in neuro-ophthalmology. Optical coherence tomography (OCT), for instance, allows high-resolution imaging of the retina and optic nerve, offering crucial information on the structural integrity of these essential components. Fundus autofluorescence imaging can provide valuable insights into retinal pathology. Magnetic resonance imaging (MRI) and functional MRI (fMRI) provide unparalleled visualization of the brain's visual pathways, enabling the detection of lesions and assessment of functional changes. Visual evoked potentials (VEPs) offer electrophysiological measures of visual pathway function, providing an additional layer of diagnostic information in subtle or atypical cases.

The spectrum of neuro-ophthalmological conditions is vast, encompassing conditions like optic neuritis, ischemic optic neuropathy, multiple sclerosis, and various compressive lesions affecting the visual pathways. Accurate diagnosis requires a careful integration of clinical findings with imaging results to determine the underlying cause and guide treatment strategies. Management often involves a multidisciplinary approach, possibly including medical treatments, surgical interventions, and rehabilitative therapies tailored to the specific nature of the condition and its impact on the patient's visual function. Understanding the interplay between the neurological and ophthalmological aspects is key to formulating effective treatment plans and achieving the best possible visual outcomes.

## 1.1 Scope and Importance

Neuro-ophthalmology stands at the crucial intersection of neurology and ophthalmology, a unique field dedicated to understanding the complex interplay between the brain and vision. Its significance lies in its ability to diagnose and treat a wide spectrum of conditions impacting sight, conditions often stemming from neurological issues affecting the visual pathways. Mastering this field allows for a more comprehensive approach to patient care, improving diagnostic accuracy and treatment efficacy. It's not simply about treating eye problems; it's about understanding how the brain interprets visual information and how disruptions in this process manifest as specific visual deficits.

The impact of neuro-ophthalmology extends far beyond the individual patient. Consider, for example, the profound effects of visual impairment on daily life. Loss of vision can lead to decreased independence, social isolation, and diminished quality of life. Neuro-ophthalmologists play a crucial role in minimizing these impacts by providing timely diagnosis and effective interventions. This proactive approach not only improves patients' lives but also reduces the significant economic burden associated with prolonged visual disability. Early detection and treatment can prevent irreversible visual loss, promoting better long-term outcomes and maximizing a patient's ability to maintain their independence.

Furthermore, this specialized field continually pushes the boundaries of medical knowledge. Advances in neuroimaging, genetic testing, and neurosurgical techniques are transforming our understanding of the visual system and opening new avenues for treatment. The insights gained through neuro-ophthalmological research contribute significantly to our broader understanding of the brain's intricate workings and provide valuable information applicable to other neurological conditions. This constant evolution ensures that future generations benefit from improved diagnostic tools and more effective therapeutic strategies. This interdisciplinary nature of the field encourages collaborative research, bringing together expertise in ophthalmology, neurology, radiology, and genetics, leading to a more comprehensive approach to understanding and treating visual dysfunction.

The scope of neuro-ophthalmology is broad, encompassing a wide range of conditions. From common disorders like optic neuritis to complex conditions affecting the visual pathways and brain structures, this specialty provides a comprehensive framework for understanding and managing the diverse array of visual problems with neurological origins. The specialist's role requires a deep understanding of both the anatomy and physiology of the visual system and the neurological principles underlying visual processing. They need to be familiar with various diagnostic tools, including advanced imaging techniques like MRI and OCT, to accurately identify the site and nature of neurological damage. Then, they use this knowledge to develop personalized treatment plans that address both the neurological and ophthalmological aspects of the patient's condition.

Ultimately, the importance of neuro-ophthalmology lies in its ability to improve the lives of those affected by neurological conditions that impact vision. By bridging the gap between neurology and ophthalmology, this specialized field offers a holistic approach to patient care, maximizing visual outcomes and improving overall quality of life. Its ongoing contributions to research and technological advancements ensures that the field will continue to evolve, offering even better diagnostic and therapeutic opportunities in the future, impacting not only vision but neurological health as a whole. This dedication to improving patients' quality of life is what makes this field so vital and rewarding. The integration of advanced imaging techniques and a deep understanding of neurological principles allows for a more accurate diagnosis and more effective treatment of often debilitating conditions. The potential for improvement in the lives of patients is truly immeasurable.

## 1.2 Historical Overview

Early observations of visual disturbances linked to neurological conditions, often anecdotal accounts from ancient civilizations, laid a rudimentary foundation. Descriptions of blindness following head trauma or strokes, though lacking the anatomical precision of modern medicine, hinted at the intricate connection between the brain and vision. These early records, scattered across various historical texts, serve as fragmented glimpses into the nascent understanding of what we now know as neuro-ophthalmology.

The Renaissance saw a gradual shift towards more systematic anatomical studies. Leonardo da Vinci's meticulous anatomical drawings, though not specifically focused on the visual pathways, contributed to a broader understanding of the human body's complexity. Later, anatomists like Vesalius, with his detailed dissections and illustrations, provided a more accurate depiction of the eye and its surrounding structures, paving the way for future research into their neurological connections. These advancements, while not directly addressing neuro-ophthalmology as a field, laid essential groundwork.

The 18th and 19th centuries witnessed significant breakthroughs in understanding the visual system. The discovery of the optic nerve's role in transmitting visual information to the brain marked a pivotal moment. Further advancements in microscopic anatomy revealed the intricate structure of the retina and the complex pathway of visual signals. Researchers began to connect specific lesions in the brain with corresponding visual impairments, establishing crucial links between neuroanatomy and visual function. These were fundamental steps, critical for neuro-ophthalmology's development.

The development of ophthalmoscopy in the mid-19th century revolutionized the field. This invention enabled clinicians to directly visualize the retina, allowing for detailed examination of its blood vessels and nerve fibers. This non-invasive diagnostic technique provided a window into the health of the visual pathway, particularly in cases of optic neuritis or other conditions affecting the retina and optic nerve. The ability to visually inspect these structures improved early diagnosis and treatment significantly. Previously inaccessible information suddenly became available, transforming the practice of ophthalmology and its intersection with neurology.

The 20th century brought about a surge in neuro-ophthalmological knowledge. Advances in neuroimaging, such as computed tomography (CT) and magnetic resonance imaging (MRI), provided unprecedented views of the brain and its structures. These technologies allowed for detailed visualization of the visual pathways, identifying lesions with greater accuracy and precision than ever before. Consequently, clinicians gained a more sophisticated understanding of the relationship between brain lesions and specific visual deficits, fueling more refined diagnostic and therapeutic approaches. This marked a transformative period, pushing forward the field's technological capabilities.

Electrophysiological studies, such as visual evoked potentials (VEPs), emerged as powerful tools for assessing the functional integrity of the visual system. These techniques allowed researchers to measure the electrical activity of the brain in response to visual stimuli. This objective assessment provided invaluable insights into the processing of visual information and the identification of functional abnormalities, complementing anatomical imaging techniques. Combining these techniques allowed for a holistic approach towards diagnosis, providing both structural and functional assessments of the visual pathways.

The latter half of the 20th century saw the rise of neuro-ophthalmology as a distinct medical subspecialty. The establishment of dedicated research programs and training fellowships helped solidify neuro-ophthalmology's position within the broader fields of neurology and ophthalmology. Collaborations between specialists and the integration of various disciplines fostered a deeper understanding of complex interactions between the visual and neurological systems, ultimately enhancing patient care. This period shaped the field into its modern form.

Today, neuro-ophthalmology continues to advance at a rapid pace. Ongoing research in areas such as genetics, molecular biology, and advanced neuroimaging techniques holds the promise of even more precise diagnostic tools and targeted therapies. Ongoing studies constantly refine our understanding of the intricate interplay between the nervous system and the visual system, pushing the boundaries of what is possible in visual function restoration and patient care. The future promises exciting advancements, building upon the substantial foundation already established.

# 2 Visual Pathways Anatomy

The retina, the light-sensitive tissue lining the back of the eye, initiates the visual journey. Photoreceptors, rods and cones, convert light into electrical signals. These signals are then transmitted via bipolar and ganglion cells, ultimately converging to form the optic nerve, a bundle of approximately one million nerve fibers. Damage to any part of this intricate structure, from the photoreceptors to the optic nerve itself, can profoundly impact vision, leading to a range of visual impairments, highlighting the critical role of the retina and optic nerve in visual acuity and overall health. Understanding their complex interplay is paramount for effective diagnosis and treatment of various eye conditions.

The optic nerve, after exiting the eye, travels toward the brain, converging at the optic chiasm, a crucial crossroads where fibers from the nasal (inner) halves of each retina cross over to the opposite side of the brain. This crossing ensures that information from the left visual field is processed by the right hemisphere, and vice versa. The optic tract, formed after the chiasm, carries these segregated visual signals to their next destination: the lateral geniculate nucleus (LGN). Lesions or anomalies at this point can manifest as characteristic visual field deficits. A thorough understanding of the optic chiasm's anatomy is, therefore, fundamental to correctly interpreting neurological visual symptoms.

The LGN, located within the thalamus, is not merely a relay station; it actively processes and refines visual information before forwarding it to the cortex. It's organized into layers, each receiving input from either the ipsilateral or contralateral eye. This layered structure is critical for binocular vision, depth perception, and color processing. Damage to the LGN can result in specific visual field losses, often involving both eyes symmetrically, showcasing its specialized role in visual processing. Moreover, the organization within the LGN itself is instrumental in understanding various neurological conditions that impact visual pathways.

From the LGN, visual signals embark on their final leg via the optic radiations, a complex network of nerve fibers projecting to the visual cortex. These radiations fan out, with different parts representing different regions of the visual field. The superior optic radiations convey information from the upper visual field, while the inferior radiations handle the lower field. Disruptions along these pathways, due to tumors, strokes, or trauma, often produce characteristic visual field defects, providing valuable clues to the location and nature of the underlying neurological lesion. Precise mapping of these pathways is crucial for neuro-ophthalmologists.

The primary visual cortex (V1), situated in the occipital lobe at the back of the brain, is the ultimate destination of visual signals. It's where conscious visual perception takes place, and it processes rudimentary aspects of vision. This area's layered structure allows for detailed analysis of visual input, including orientation, motion, and color. Damage to V1 can lead to cortical blindness, a complete loss of vision in the corresponding part of the visual field, emphasizing its fundamental role in visual perception. The complexities of V1 structure and function continue to be areas of intensive study. Further processing then occurs in extrastriate areas V2, V3, and so forth, responsible for progressively higher-level visual processing, including object recognition and spatial awareness. Understanding the visual processing cascade that begins in the retina and ends in the visual cortex requires mastery of this anatomical complexity.

## 2.1 Retina and Optic Nerve

The retina, a marvel of biological engineering, lines the back of the eye. Millions of photoreceptor cells, rods for low-light vision and cones for color and detail, meticulously translate light into electrical signals. These signals, the very foundation of our visual perception, initiate an intricate journey. The meticulous arrangement of these cells, their precise connections, and the layers that process and relay the information are crucial for healthy vision. Damage to any part of this intricate structure can severely impair sight, highlighting the sensitivity and importance of this initial stage of visual processing.

Consider the optic nerve, a bundle of over a million nerve fibers emerging from the retina. This crucial pathway transmits visual information from the eye to the brain. Its structure, a tightly packed collection of axons, ensures efficient signal transmission. The myelin sheath, a fatty insulating layer surrounding these axons, facilitates rapid conduction. Any disruption to this sheath, or damage to the nerve fibers themselves, dramatically impairs the speed and accuracy of signal transmission leading to a cascade of visual problems. This simple anatomical structure underpins the complexity of our vision, its delicate balance vulnerable to various diseases and traumas.

The vascular supply to both retina and optic nerve is equally critical. The central retinal artery, a branch of the ophthalmic artery, nourishes the inner layers of the retina, delivering oxygen and nutrients essential for its function. The choroidal circulation supplies the outer layers, providing the metabolic support for photoreceptor function. Compromise in either system, whether due to blockage, inflammation, or other vascular issues, results in immediate disruption of visual processing. This vulnerability highlights the importance of cardiovascular health in maintaining eye health. A healthy circulatory system is crucial for the sustained functionality of the delicate retinal and optic nerve tissues. This often-overlooked connection underscores the holistic approach needed in neuro-ophthalmology.

Understanding the anatomy of the retina and optic nerve is fundamental to diagnosing and managing neuro-ophthalmological conditions. Detailed knowledge of retinal layers, photoreceptor types, and the precise arrangement of nerve fibers in the optic nerve is crucial for interpreting ophthalmological findings. This understanding forms the bedrock of clinical practice, informing diagnostic strategies and guiding therapeutic choices. It allows the practitioner to better correlate anatomical findings with the patient's visual symptoms and provide accurate diagnoses, and this precise understanding ultimately impacts the choice of intervention.

Visual field testing, a cornerstone of neuro-ophthalmological examination, reveals the functional integrity of the visual pathways. Detecting scotomas (blind spots), peripheral vision loss, or other visual field defects provides valuable clues about the location and nature of the lesion along the visual pathway. By mapping these defects, clinicians pinpoint the affected area, whether it be the retina, optic nerve, or a more central region. The specific pattern of visual field loss often helps differentiate between different pathologies, providing crucial diagnostic information for targeted management strategies. Combining this information with detailed anatomical knowledge allows clinicians to create the most effective and personalized treatment plans.

Damage to the retina or optic nerve manifests in various ways, depending on the location and extent of the injury. This damage may result from a number of etiologies, from trauma to vascular events, inflammatory processes to degenerative diseases. The presentation can range from subtle visual distortions to complete blindness. Acute events, such as optic neuritis or retinal artery occlusion, may present with sudden vision loss. Chronic conditions, like glaucoma or age-related macular degeneration, often cause gradual, progressive deterioration of vision. This requires a careful and comprehensive evaluation. A good history and physical examination paired with advanced imaging techniques provide a complete clinical picture which helps in developing an effective therapeutic approach.

In summary, the retina and optic nerve represent the initial and crucial stages of visual signal transmission. Their complex anatomy, intricate vascular supply, and vulnerability to various pathologies underscore the importance of a thorough understanding of their structure and function. This detailed knowledge is essential for the accurate diagnosis and management of a wide spectrum of neuro-ophthalmological conditions. A deep understanding of the intricate workings of the retina and optic nerve allows neuro-ophthalmologists to deliver the best possible care for patients experiencing visual impairments. The precision and thoroughness demanded in this field make it truly rewarding and meaningful. Through meticulous examination and advanced technologies, we continually refine our understanding of these vital structures, leading to improved outcomes for our patients.

## 2.2 Optic Chiasm and Tract

The optic chiasm, a crucial structure nestled at the base of the brain, is where the optic nerves from each eye meet and partially cross. Imagine it as a vital crossroads, where half of the nerve fibers from each eye switch sides, a fascinating anatomical arrangement that's fundamental to our binocular vision. This decussation, the crossing over, ensures that information from the right visual field of both eyes is processed by the left side of the brain, and vice versa. Understanding this intricate process is essential for diagnosing and managing a wide range of neuro-ophthalmological conditions.

This crossing isn't random; it's precisely organized. Nasal retinal fibers—those originating from the inner half of the retina—cross at the chiasm, while temporal fibers—from the outer half—continue ipsilaterally, remaining on the same side of the brain. This precise arrangement allows for the creation of a complete representation of the visual world in each hemisphere of the brain. Consider the implications if this were disrupted; the consequences for visual perception would be profound.

Moving beyond the chiasm, the optic tracts emerge, carrying the now partially decussated fibers. These tracts are not simply conduits; they are complex pathways relaying visual information. They curve gracefully around the midbrain, their trajectory crucial for understanding visual field defects that can stem from lesions along their route. Damage to the optic tract, for example, will typically produce a contralateral homonymous hemianopia—loss of vision in the same half of the visual field in both eyes on the opposite side of the brain lesion.

The anatomy of the optic tract is surprisingly complex. It's not just a uniform bundle of fibers; its organization reflects the retinotopic mapping of the visual field. Different parts of the tract carry information from specific regions of the retina, mirroring the spatial organization of the visual world. This retinotopic organization continues into the lateral geniculate nucleus (LGN), maintaining the spatial relationships critical for accurate visual perception. Therefore, lesions at specific points along the optic tract can cause very specific visual field defects.

A detailed understanding of the optic tract's anatomy is paramount for interpreting visual field defects. For instance, a lesion affecting only a portion of the optic tract will create a corresponding, sectorial scotoma in the contralateral visual field. These sectorial defects are telling; they provide important clues to the lesion's location and size. A complete understanding of the optic tract's complex organization is essential for accurate diagnosis.

Think of it this way: the optic tract is not simply a wire carrying electrical signals; it's a sophisticated information highway, with designated lanes for different types of visual information. Studying its structure, and the precise organization of its fibers, is crucial for neuro-ophthalmologists to fully understand how the visual system processes and interprets the world around us. The arrangement of the fibers isn't merely anatomical; it's functional, underpinning the remarkable ability of the brain to construct a coherent visual experience.

Clinically, understanding the optic chiasm and tract's anatomy is crucial for diagnosing and localizing lesions. Visual field testing, in conjunction with neuroimaging, allows clinicians to precisely identify the location and extent of damage to these critical structures. Lesions at the chiasm, for instance, often cause bitemporal hemianopia—loss of the temporal (outer) visual fields in both eyes—a hallmark sign of chiasmal compression.

Furthermore, detailed knowledge of the optic pathways' intricate organization aids in differential diagnosis. Differentiating between a lesion in the optic nerve, chiasm, or tract requires careful assessment of the visual field defects and correlation with neuroimaging findings. For instance, a lesion in the optic nerve will generally cause a monocular visual field loss, while a lesion in the optic tract will typically result in a contralateral homonymous hemianopia. These distinctions are critical for guiding appropriate management.

This knowledge is not solely confined to theoretical understanding. It has significant implications for patient care. Precise localization of lesions through understanding of the optic chiasm and tract helps determine appropriate therapeutic interventions, whether medical or surgical. Early diagnosis and accurate localization, enabled by a strong understanding of these structures' anatomy and function, lead to improved patient outcomes and a better quality of life. The finer points of this anatomy are crucial for navigating this complex field.

The study of the optic chiasm and tract goes beyond simply memorizing anatomical structures. It's about appreciating the intricate interplay between form and function. This chapter has been aimed at providing foundational knowledge and an understanding of its importance. This fundamental knowledge underpins neuro-ophthalmological practice. Grasping the intricacies of this critical part of the visual pathway equips the clinician with the tools for precise diagnosis and effective management of a wide array of neuro-ophthalmological conditions. Mastering this area is essential for the successful practice of neuro-ophthalmology.

## 2.3 Lateral Geniculate Nucleus

The lateral geniculate nucleus (LGN), a crucial relay station within the thalamus, plays a pivotal role in visual processing. Imagine it as a sophisticated sorting office, meticulously organizing and refining the raw visual data received from the retina before forwarding it to the visual cortex. Its layered structure, six distinct layers to be precise, each with specific functional properties, is key to understanding its complex role. Parvocellular layers, for instance, primarily handle fine detail and color perception, while magnocellular layers focus on motion detection and overall luminance. This layered architecture allows for parallel processing of visual information, a highly efficient system enhancing our visual experience.

Understanding the LGN's function goes beyond simple signal transmission. It actively participates in shaping visual perception. Studies suggest that the LGN modulates information flow based on factors such as attention and context. It isn't just a passive conduit; it actively filters and enhances certain aspects of the visual signal, contributing to our perception of contrast, brightness, and depth. This active role highlights the complexity of visual processing and the importance of the LGN as more than a mere relay.

Clinically, the LGN's significance is undeniable. Lesions affecting the LGN can lead to a variety of visual disturbances, often manifesting as visual field deficits. These deficits aren't always uniform; they can be highly specific depending on which layers are damaged. A lesion affecting the parvocellular layers might primarily affect color vision, while damage to magnocellular layers could result in deficits in motion perception. Such precise correlations between anatomical location and visual dysfunction underscore the LGN's importance in clinical neuro-ophthalmology.

Diagnosing LGN lesions requires advanced imaging techniques. High-resolution MRI scans can sometimes reveal structural abnormalities within the LGN, providing direct evidence of pathology. Functional MRI (fMRI) offers a more dynamic perspective, allowing clinicians to assess the LGN's activity during visual tasks. By comparing the activity patterns in a patient's LGN to those of a healthy control group, subtle functional impairments might be detected even in the absence of obvious structural changes. This emphasizes the combined use of structural and functional techniques for accurate diagnosis.

Furthermore, the interaction between the LGN and other brain regions is equally crucial. The LGN doesn't operate in isolation; it receives input from various brain areas, including the brainstem and the visual cortex itself. These feedback connections allow for top-down modulation of visual processing, influencing what we perceive and how we interpret visual information. Understanding these complex interactions provides a more complete picture of how the visual system operates as a dynamic network rather than a series of isolated modules.

The LGN's role in visual processing extends beyond basic sensory input. It actively participates in higher-order visual functions, such as object recognition and spatial awareness. By integrating information from various sources and refining it based on contextual clues, the LGN contributes to our ability to make sense of the visual world. This is critical for everyday tasks involving visual navigation and object interaction.

Research continues to unravel the intricacies of the LGN's function. Scientists are exploring its role in visual plasticity, the brain's ability to adapt to changes in visual input. Understanding this adaptability is crucial for developing effective therapies for visual impairments. Moreover, ongoing research focuses on understanding the LGN's involvement in conditions like amblyopia and visual agnosia. These investigations shed light on the role of the LGN in both normal and abnormal visual development.

In conclusion, the lateral geniculate nucleus represents a critical node in the visual pathway. Its intricate layered structure, active participation in shaping visual perception, and susceptibility to lesions that result in distinctive visual field deficits make it a key focus for neuro-ophthalmologists. Advanced imaging techniques are vital for evaluating both structural and functional integrity. Understanding its complex interactions with other brain regions and ongoing research into its role in visual plasticity provide a holistic perspective on the LGN's significance and its impact on our daily visual experiences. This understanding is fundamental to improving the diagnosis and treatment of visual disorders.

## 2.4 Optic Radiations

The optic radiations, a crucial component of the visual pathway, are a complex system of nerve fibers that relay visual information from the lateral geniculate nucleus (LGN) to the visual cortex. Understanding their intricate anatomy and function is paramount for diagnosing and managing a wide range of neuro-ophthalmological conditions. These fibers, fanning out like the spokes of a wheel, are not simply a direct conduit; their organization is highly structured, with distinct pathways carrying information from specific retinal regions. Damage to these pathways, often resulting from stroke, trauma, or tumors, leads to characteristic visual field defects that provide invaluable diagnostic clues.

Consider, for instance, the Meyer's loop, a portion of the optic radiation that curves around the temporal horn of the lateral ventricle. Lesions affecting this loop, such as a stroke in the temporal lobe, typically cause a superior quadrantanopia, a loss of vision in the upper quadrant of the visual field in the contralateral eye. This precise correspondence between anatomical location and visual field deficit is a cornerstone of neuro-ophthalmological diagnosis. We can use this knowledge to pinpoint the precise location of the damage.

Conversely, damage to the dorsal optic radiation, running superiorly through the parietal lobe, results in a different pattern of visual field loss – an inferior quadrantanopia. Clinicians must carefully analyze the specific visual field defects to determine the location and extent of damage within the optic radiations. A thorough understanding of the anatomy of the optic radiations is essential for accurate interpretation. This is critical for effective treatment planning.

The diagnostic process often relies on a combination of techniques. Visual field testing, which maps the extent of visual field loss, provides crucial information about the potential site of lesion. High-resolution neuroimaging techniques, such as MRI, can pinpoint the location and size of the lesion in relation to the anatomical structures of the optic radiations, confirming the clinical findings from the visual field exam. Advanced imaging can reveal subtle lesions invisible on simpler examination methods. This provides an invaluable tool for better precision and less invasive methods.

Moreover, the complexity of the optic radiations extends beyond their anatomical organization. Their functional organization reflects the intricate processing of visual information. Different parts of the optic radiations might process specific aspects of visual information, such as color, motion, or form. Damage to specific regions within the radiations might lead to a selective impairment of these aspects of vision. Understanding these functional aspects is critical for a complete understanding of the visual system.

For example, some individuals might experience difficulty with object recognition or face processing (prosopagnosia) following damage to specific portions of the optic radiations and associated visual cortical regions. This goes beyond simple visual field loss, highlighting the nuanced nature of visual processing and the complexity of the optic radiations. These subtleties are often overlooked without deep knowledge of the underlying neuroanatomy.

Therefore, mastering the anatomy and functional organization of the optic radiations is fundamental to the neuro-ophthalmologist's practice. By carefully analyzing the patient's visual field defects, combined with advanced neuroimaging techniques, we can accurately pinpoint the location and extent of lesions within these crucial pathways. This detailed understanding guides therapeutic strategies, allowing for better patient outcomes. Understanding the optic radiations is key to improving patient care. This detailed approach ensures a thorough diagnostic workup.

Accurate diagnosis enables targeted treatment strategies. In cases of vascular lesions, for example, the location of the lesion within the optic radiations will directly influence treatment choices. Furthermore, knowledge of the affected area facilitates the selection of appropriate rehabilitative therapies. Patients with optic radiation lesions can benefit from specific visual rehabilitation exercises aimed at improving residual visual function. This approach is more targeted than general rehabilitation programs.

Finally, ongoing research continues to shed light on the subtle complexities of the optic radiations. Advancements in neuroimaging and functional brain mapping technologies are leading to a more refined understanding of their functional organization and the specific roles different parts play in visual processing. This evolving knowledge will continue to enhance our ability to diagnose and treat conditions affecting the visual pathways. The more we understand, the better we can help.

## 2.5 Visual Cortex

The visual cortex, located in the occipital lobe at the rear of the brain, isn't a single, monolithic structure; rather, it's a complex network of areas, each specialized for different aspects of visual processing. Think of it as a sophisticated assembly line, where raw visual data undergoes a series of transformations, ultimately resulting in our conscious perception of the world. This intricate system allows us to discern shapes, colors, movement, and depth, all crucial for navigating our environment.

Understanding the visual cortex is vital in neuro-ophthalmology because damage to any part of this network can lead to a variety of visual impairments. Consider a stroke affecting a specific region; the resulting visual deficit will depend on the precise location and extent of the damage. This highlights the importance of precise neuroimaging techniques, allowing clinicians to pinpoint the affected area for accurate diagnosis and treatment planning.

Different parts of the visual cortex perform distinct roles. V1, or the primary visual cortex, receives direct input from the lateral geniculate nucleus, initiating the process of visual interpretation. It analyzes basic visual features like lines, edges, and orientations, the building blocks of visual perception. Further processing occurs in extrastriate areas, like V2, V4, and V5, which are responsible for more complex aspects such as color perception, shape recognition, and motion detection.

Damage to V1, for instance, can result in cortical blindness, a condition where individuals may have perfectly healthy eyes and optic nerves but are unable to consciously see. This stark contrast emphasizes the crucial role of the visual cortex in visual awareness. It is not merely a relay station but the place where raw sensory data is transformed into meaningful visual experience. Other lesions in the extrastriate areas can cause more specific visual deficits such as achromatopsia (color blindness) or akinetopsia (motion blindness). The precise nature of the visual disturbance can help localize the damage within the visual cortex.

To diagnose visual cortex disorders, advanced imaging techniques are crucial. Functional MRI (fMRI) allows visualization of brain activity, revealing which areas are involved in specific visual tasks. This provides a non-invasive way to assess the functional integrity of the visual cortex, complementing structural imaging such as MRI, which shows anatomical details. Such techniques are essential for differentiating between different types of visual deficits, guiding treatment strategies, and monitoring recovery. Careful examination of visual field defects, often mapped through perimetry, provides critical information that correlates with lesion location.

Treatment options for visual cortex damage vary considerably depending on the underlying cause and the severity of the deficit. While there's no cure for damage to the visual cortex itself, rehabilitation therapies can be incredibly beneficial. These therapies aim to improve visual function through targeted exercises and strategies that help the brain adapt and compensate for the damage. They might involve visual stimulation or training focused on specific visual skills, such as object recognition or spatial awareness. Early intervention is key.

The visual cortex is more than just a passive receiver of visual information. It's a dynamic and adaptable system capable of remarkable plasticity, meaning it can reorganize and adapt to changes and injuries. This neuroplasticity is the foundation for rehabilitation efforts. The brain's ability to rewire itself underscores the potential for recovery, even after significant visual cortex damage. By understanding the functional organization and plasticity of the visual cortex, clinicians can develop more effective treatment strategies and improve the quality of life for individuals with visual impairments.

Research continues to unravel the intricate workings of the visual cortex, continuously revealing the complexity of visual perception and its neurological underpinnings. Advancements in neuroimaging and our deepening understanding of brain plasticity offer hope for improved diagnostic techniques and more effective therapies in the future. The continuing exploration of this fascinating area of the brain promises further advancements in the care and treatment of those with visual impairments. This understanding is absolutely pivotal to neuro-ophthalmology.

# 3 Common Neuro-Ophthalmological Conditions

Optic neuritis, an inflammatory condition affecting the optic nerve, often presents with sudden, unilateral vision loss, typically described as blurry or foggy. Pain, especially with eye movement, is a common symptom, further distinguishing it from other causes of vision impairment. The condition's etiology is diverse, ranging from autoimmune diseases like multiple sclerosis to infections and even certain medications. Diagnosing optic neuritis involves a thorough neurological and ophthalmological examination, including visual acuity testing, visual field assessment, and optical coherence tomography (OCT) to evaluate optic nerve structure. Magnetic resonance imaging (MRI) of the brain and orbits may be necessary to rule out other conditions, particularly multiple sclerosis. Treatment typically involves corticosteroids, aiming to reduce inflammation and potentially improve visual recovery. Early intervention is crucial for optimal outcomes, emphasizing the importance of prompt diagnosis and management.

Ischemic optic neuropathy, on the other hand, results from reduced blood flow to the optic nerve head. This leads to damage of the nerve fibers, consequently affecting vision. The condition is primarily divided into two types: anterior ischemic optic neuropathy (AION), which affects the anterior part of the optic nerve, and posterior ischemic optic neuropathy (PION), impacting the posterior section. AION, more prevalent in older individuals, often presents with painless, unilateral vision loss, with the acuity of the affected eye being severely diminished. Risk factors for AION include hypertension, diabetes, and sleep apnea. PION, in contrast, is associated with systemic illnesses and vascular conditions that impair blood supply to the optic nerve. Diagnosis relies heavily on clinical findings, visual field testing, and OCT, revealing the characteristic structural changes in the optic nerve head. Treatment for ischemic optic neuropathy focuses on managing underlying risk factors and potentially improving blood flow. While visual recovery may be limited, management focuses on optimizing the remaining vision and preventing further damage.

Understanding the distinctions between these two conditions is vital for appropriate management. Although both involve optic nerve dysfunction and vision loss, their causes, presentations, and potential treatments differ significantly. The clinical picture, including the presence or absence of pain, visual field deficits, and the patient's overall health status, directs the diagnostic process. Imaging techniques, such as OCT and MRI, provide critical objective evidence to confirm the diagnosis and guide treatment strategies. Early intervention is key in both cases, aiming to minimize the extent of vision loss and optimize visual function. In practice, a neuro-ophthalmologist's expertise is invaluable in differentiating these conditions and creating a tailored management plan.

The importance of a comprehensive evaluation cannot be overstated. Detailed patient history, including the onset and character of visual symptoms, associated medical conditions, and medication use, is essential in guiding differential diagnosis. This is further amplified by the detailed ophthalmological examination that assesses visual acuity, pupil responses, and ocular motility. Furthermore, careful visual field analysis identifies the specific areas of vision impairment. This thorough approach aids in differentiating optic neuritis from ischemic optic neuropathy, as well as from other neuro-ophthalmological conditions such as glaucoma or optic nerve tumors. Collaboration between ophthalmologists and neurologists ensures a comprehensive assessment and coordinated management plan, ultimately improving patient outcomes. Remember that a proper diagnosis is critical in selecting effective therapeutic interventions.

Moreover, managing expectations is a crucial aspect of patient care. While treatment aims to improve visual function, recovery varies widely among individuals. Factors such as the severity of the condition, the time elapsed since onset of symptoms, and the presence of underlying medical conditions all influence the prognosis. Open and honest communication between the healthcare provider and patient regarding the likely trajectory of the disease, potential complications, and realistic goals of treatment is paramount. This collaborative approach fosters a sense of understanding and empowers patients to actively participate in their care, improving adherence to treatment plans and potentially enhancing the quality of their lives, even with vision loss. The focus should always be on maximizing functional vision and improving quality of life.

## 3.1 Optic Neuritis

Optic neuritis, an inflammatory process affecting the optic nerve, presents a challenging clinical picture. Its hallmark is a sudden, often unilateral, loss of vision, typically accompanied by pain, particularly with eye movements. This pain distinguishes it from many other causes of vision loss, providing a crucial diagnostic clue. The acuity of vision loss can vary dramatically, from a mild blurring to complete blindness. Prompt diagnosis and treatment are essential to minimize permanent vision loss and improve the patient's prognosis.

Early diagnosis hinges on a thorough clinical examination, encompassing visual acuity testing, color vision assessment, and a meticulous visual field analysis. A careful ophthalmoscopic evaluation may reveal subtle swelling or pallor of the optic disc, though these findings are not always present, particularly in early stages. Magnetic resonance imaging (MRI) scans are frequently employed, not only to confirm the diagnosis but also to identify the underlying cause and extent of inflammation. MRI's sensitivity in detecting optic nerve inflammation is superior to other imaging modalities.

The etiology of optic neuritis is multifaceted. In many cases, it's associated with autoimmune disorders, most notably multiple sclerosis (MS). In fact, optic neuritis serves as a significant risk factor and potential early manifestation of MS. Other possible causes include infections (viral or bacterial), certain medications, and less common conditions like sarcoidosis. A comprehensive history, including inquiries into prior illnesses and medications, is paramount in identifying these potential risk factors. The patient's neurological examination plays a vital role in confirming this diagnosis and guiding appropriate treatment, with specific focus on any other neurological symptoms present.

Treatment strategies are tailored to the severity of the optic neuritis and underlying cause. In most cases, high-dose intravenous corticosteroids are the mainstay of treatment, aimed at rapidly reducing inflammation and improving visual outcomes. Oral corticosteroids may be used subsequently to maintain remission and prevent relapse. The duration and specific regimen of corticosteroid therapy are determined on a case-by-case basis, considering factors such as the patient's overall health and the severity of their vision loss.

Beyond corticosteroids, the management of optic neuritis frequently involves addressing any underlying autoimmune condition that might be contributing to its development. For instance, patients with MS often require long-term disease-modifying therapies to manage their underlying neurological disorder. Careful patient monitoring and close collaboration between neurologists and ophthalmologists is essential for the best outcome, and these specialists may work together using a multidisciplinary approach.

The prognosis for optic neuritis varies depending on several factors, including the severity of the initial visual loss, the presence of underlying disease, and the promptness of treatment. While most patients experience some degree of visual recovery, complete restoration of vision is not always guaranteed. Visual recovery often occurs gradually over several weeks or months, and the potential for relapses always exists, especially in those individuals with MS. Rehabilitation of vision in the cases with incomplete recovery is crucial. Regular follow-up examinations are vital to monitor visual function and address any potential complications.

In summary, optic neuritis presents a spectrum of challenges, demanding a thorough investigation and a comprehensive treatment strategy. The collaboration between ophthalmology and neurology proves essential in managing this condition effectively. Early identification and intervention are key to improving patient outcomes and minimizing the long-term impact on vision.

## 3.2 Ischemic Optic Neuropathy

Ischemic optic neuropathy (ION) is a serious condition affecting the optic nerve's blood supply, leading to vision loss. Understanding its nuances is crucial for timely diagnosis and management. This chapter focuses on the two main types: anterior ION (AION) and posterior ION (PION).

AION, more common, typically affects individuals over 50, often with underlying vascular risk factors like hypertension, diabetes, or hyperlipidemia. The sudden, painless loss of vision is its hallmark symptom, usually unilateral. It's often described as a "curtain coming down" over the affected eye. The severity varies; some experience a mild decrease in visual acuity, while others suffer near-total blindness. Diagnosis often relies on ophthalmoscopic findings revealing swelling of the optic disc, often pale and exhibiting splinter hemorrhages. Fluorescein angiography can help visualize the impaired blood flow.

PION, in contrast, is less common and presents differently. It frequently affects younger individuals, often associated with giant cell arteritis (GCA), a serious inflammatory condition. In these cases, the vision loss might be accompanied by headaches, jaw claudication, and other systemic symptoms. PION's clinical presentation may include a more subtle swelling of the optic disc, and angiography may show abnormalities in the posterior ciliary arteries. It's crucial to remember that prompt diagnosis and treatment of GCA are paramount to prevent blindness in the fellow eye. Early recognition of GCA requires a high index of suspicion in patients presenting with PION symptoms, coupled with elevated inflammatory markers and temporal artery biopsy. Effective management of ION begins with careful assessment of risk factors and a thorough ophthalmological examination. For AION, the focus is primarily on managing underlying conditions like hypertension and diabetes, thus minimizing further vascular damage. There's no proven treatment to reverse the vision loss already incurred; however, controlling vascular risk factors is key to preserving remaining vision and preventing bilateral involvement. Regular monitoring of visual acuity and visual field testing are essential.

The treatment approach for PION differs significantly, requiring immediate and aggressive intervention. GCA is a medical emergency that demands prompt treatment with high-dose corticosteroids to suppress inflammation and prevent further optic nerve damage. Rapid diagnosis and initiation of corticosteroids are vital to preserve remaining vision and reduce the risk of blindness in the contralateral eye. Long-term management includes monitoring for GCA recurrence and careful assessment for potential side effects of corticosteroid therapy.

Differential diagnosis is critical in ION cases, ruling out other conditions like optic neuritis, compressive lesions, and other forms of ischemic optic neuropathy. The patient's age, history of vascular disease, presence of systemic symptoms, and specific ophthalmoscopic findings are all vital clues in making an accurate diagnosis. Imaging studies such as MRI or CT scans may be necessary to rule out underlying causes like compressive lesions or tumors that mimic the symptoms of ION.

Beyond immediate medical management, rehabilitation strategies play a significant role in improving patients' quality of life. Low-vision aids, such as magnifying glasses or electronic devices, can help patients adapt to their vision loss. Occupational therapy can help patients learn new strategies to navigate their daily activities and maintain independence. Psychological support is equally important to help patients cope with the emotional challenges associated with visual impairment. Support groups can provide a sense of community and shared experi-

ence, facilitating the adaptation process.
In conclusion, understanding the various subtypes of ION, their underlying causes, and appropriate management strategies is paramount for neuro-ophthalmologists. A detailed patient history, thorough ophthalmological examination, and appropriate investigations are essential to arrive at an accurate diagnosis and initiate timely intervention. The multidisciplinary approach, involving ophthalmologists, neurologists, and other specialists, is crucial in delivering the best possible outcomes for patients suffering from this challenging condition. The focus should always be on mitigating the underlying risk factors, controlling inflammation (if present), and providing support to enhance the patients' adaptation to their vision loss. The future may bring further advancements in understanding the pathophysiology and developing more effective treatments for ION. Early detection and prompt management remain crucial for preserving vision and improving patient outcomes.

# 4 Advanced Imaging Techniques

Optical coherence tomography (OCT) offers high-resolution cross-sectional imaging of the retina and optic nerve, revealing subtle structural changes often missed by traditional ophthalmoscopy. Its ability to quantify retinal nerve fiber layer thickness is particularly valuable in monitoring disease progression in conditions like glaucoma and optic neuritis, providing objective measures of neurodegeneration. Furthermore, OCT angiography, a newer technique, allows visualization of retinal and choroidal vasculature, offering insights into microvascular abnormalities that may contribute to visual impairment. This non-invasive procedure proves invaluable in the early detection and management of various neuro-ophthalmological disorders.

Fundus autofluorescence (FAF) imaging provides a complementary approach, visualizing the distribution of lipofuscin, a fluorescent pigment accumulating in retinal pigment epithelium (RPE) cells with age and disease. Abnormal patterns of FAF can indicate dysfunction or damage to the RPE, crucial for maintaining retinal health. For instance, in age-related macular degeneration (AMD), FAF highlights areas of RPE atrophy and hyperautofluorescence, aiding in disease staging and treatment planning. Combining FAF with OCT enhances diagnostic accuracy, allowing for a more comprehensive assessment of retinal structure and function. Its use is expanding to other neuro-ophthalmological conditions where RPE involvement is suspected.

Magnetic resonance imaging (MRI) is indispensable for evaluating the brain and visual pathways, providing detailed anatomical information about the optic nerves, chiasm, tracts, and occipital lobes. High-resolution T1-weighted and T2-weighted images can detect lesions, inflammation, or atrophy affecting these structures. Diffusion tensor imaging (DTI), a specialized MRI technique, measures the diffusion of water molecules within white matter tracts, quantifying the integrity of the visual pathways. This is particularly useful in assessing optic nerve damage in various neurological conditions. MRI has proven incredibly valuable, enabling precise localization and characterization of lesions.

Functional MRI (fMRI) goes a step further, measuring brain activity indirectly by detecting changes in blood flow. By presenting visual stimuli to the patient during fMRI scanning, we can map the areas of the visual cortex activated by specific visual tasks. This functional information complements the anatomical data provided by structural MRI. fMRI is particularly useful in assessing functional deficits resulting from lesions within the visual pathways. Identifying areas of disrupted visual processing guides clinicians in prognosis and intervention strategies. These images provide important information for treatment decisions.

Visual evoked potentials (VEPs) are electrophysiological tests that measure the electrical activity in the visual cortex in response to visual stimuli. By analyzing the latency and amplitude of these evoked potentials, we can assess the integrity and speed of visual signal transmission along the visual pathways. VEPs are particularly sensitive to demyelinating lesions affecting the optic nerves, as seen in multiple sclerosis. They offer a non-invasive method of evaluating visual pathway function, complementing anatomical imaging techniques such as MRI. The results of VEPs, particularly the latency measurements, offer valuable insights.

The integration of these advanced imaging techniques significantly enhances our ability to diagnose, monitor, and manage neuro-ophthalmological conditions. OCT provides high-resolution retinal imaging, FAF reveals RPE dysfunction, MRI assesses the integrity of the visual pathways, fMRI maps functional activity in the visual cortex, and VEPs assess the speed of visual signal transmission. The combined use of these techniques allows for a comprehensive evaluation of both structural and functional aspects of the visual system, leading to more accurate diagnoses and more effective treatment strategies. This multifaceted approach is crucial for optimizing visual outcomes for patients with neuro-ophthalmological diseases. The synergistic use of these techniques is revolutionizing the field.

## 4.1 OCT and Fundus Autofluorescence

Optical coherence tomography (OCT) offers a high-resolution, cross-sectional view of retinal structures, providing invaluable information about retinal nerve fiber layer thickness, macular morphology, and the presence of inner retinal abnormalities. This non-invasive technique allows for detailed assessment of the structural integrity of the retina, which is crucial in various neuro-ophthalmological conditions. For example, in optic neuritis, OCT can reveal characteristic thinning of the retinal nerve fiber layer, correlating with the severity of the disease and potentially aiding in prognosis.

Fundus autofluorescence (FAF) imaging, on the other hand, reveals the distribution of lipofuscin, a metabolic byproduct accumulating in retinal pigment epithelium (RPE) cells. Changes in autofluorescence patterns can indicate dysfunction within the RPE, a critical component of the outer retina. Areas of increased or decreased autofluorescence can highlight areas of RPE stress, atrophy, or degeneration, often preceding clinically apparent structural changes detectable by OCT. Combining FAF with OCT allows for a more comprehensive evaluation of retinal health.

The integration of OCT and FAF is particularly beneficial in the diagnosis and management of several conditions. For instance, in age-related macular degeneration (AMD), OCT helps visualize structural changes like drusen formation and geographic atrophy, while FAF provides insight into the metabolic activity and stress of the RPE. Early detection of these changes is crucial for timely intervention and potentially slow-

ing disease progression. Similarly, in various inherited retinal dystrophies, FAF can reveal characteristic patterns of hyper\item and hypo-autofluorescence, helping to differentiate between various subtypes.
Think of OCT and FAF as complementary tools, each providing a unique perspective on retinal health. OCT provides the structural blueprint, highlighting architectural changes, while FAF unveils the metabolic landscape, reflecting the functional status of the retina. Therefore, a combined approach offers a more holistic understanding than either technique alone. Their combined use enhances diagnostic accuracy and allows for more personalized management strategies.
Furthermore, the use of these imaging techniques is not limited to diagnosis. They can also monitor disease progression and treatment response. Serial OCT and FAF imaging can track changes in retinal structure and function over time, providing valuable information for assessing the efficacy of therapies. This longitudinal monitoring is particularly important in conditions where early intervention is critical for preserving vision.
Consider a patient presenting with unexplained vision loss. Initial clinical examination may not reveal a definitive diagnosis. However, OCT scans may show thinning of the retinal nerve fiber layer suggestive of optic neuropathy, while FAF might display areas of RPE dysfunction. Together, these findings can guide further investigations and aid in reaching a precise diagnosis.
The practical application extends beyond the clinical setting. Research utilizing OCT and FAF has significantly advanced our understanding of retinal diseases, contributing to the development of novel diagnostic and therapeutic approaches. By enabling detailed visualization of retinal alterations, these techniques have accelerated the progress of clinical trials and the development of personalized treatment strategies. This ongoing research makes it clear that proficiency in interpreting these images is not merely a technical skill, but an essential aspect of modern neuro-ophthalmological practice.
In summary, mastering the interpretation of OCT and FAF images is an essential skill for any neuro-ophthalmologist. The combined use of these techniques significantly enhances diagnostic accuracy and en-

ables comprehensive monitoring of retinal diseases. Their combined power lies in their ability to provide both structural and functional information, creating a more complete picture of the retina's health and disease processes. The integration of these advanced imaging methods into clinical practice has revolutionized our approach to neuro-ophthalmological conditions, improving both diagnosis and patient care. The development and refinement of this technology is ongoing, ensuring the future of neuro-ophthalmology relies heavily on the appropriate and effective use of OCT and FAF imaging for diagnosis and disease monitoring. This is crucial in making informed decisions about treatment and management plans for patients with various neuro-ophthalmological disorders.

## 4.2 MRI and fMRI of Visual Pathways

Magnetic resonance imaging (MRI) provides exquisite anatomical detail of the visual pathways, allowing for the identification of lesions and structural abnormalities that might otherwise go undetected. We can visualize the optic nerves, chiasm, tracts, lateral geniculate nuclei, and optic radiations with remarkable clarity, revealing subtle changes in size, shape, or signal intensity that are indicative of pathology. For instance, an optic neuritis might present as an area of increased signal intensity on T2-weighted images, reflecting inflammation and edema within the nerve. Similarly, compressive lesions, such as tumors, can be identified by their mass effect on adjacent structures. The precise location and extent of the lesion are crucial for guiding treatment strategies and predicting prognosis.

Functional MRI (fMRI), in contrast, allows us to visualize brain activity during visual tasks. This technique measures changes in blood flow and oxygenation, providing a map of brain regions involved in visual processing. By having a patient perform specific visual tasks, like identifying objects or tracking moving stimuli, we can assess the functional integrity of different parts of the visual pathway. For example, a lesion affecting the occipital lobe might show decreased activation in the corresponding visual cortex area during visual stimulation. This functional information complements the structural data obtained from standard MRI, providing a more complete picture of the patient's visual system. It's essential to note, however, that fMRI is highly sensitive to motion artifacts, meaning patient cooperation is crucial for obtaining high-quality data.

The combination of structural MRI and fMRI offers a powerful approach to investigating neuro-ophthalmological disorders. By integrating these two modalities, clinicians can obtain a comprehensive understanding of both the anatomical and functional consequences of lesions within the visual pathways. This multimodal approach facilitates more accurate diagnosis, improved prognosis prediction, and personalized treatment planning. For example, a patient presenting with visual field deficits might undergo both structural MRI to identify the location of a lesion and fMRI to assess the extent of functional impairment. This information then helps guide treatment choices, whether it involves medication, surgery, or rehabilitative therapy.

Consider a patient suspected of having multiple sclerosis. Structural MRI might reveal scattered lesions throughout the brain and spinal cord, including some affecting the optic nerves. To further assess the impact of these lesions on visual processing, fMRI can be used to assess the responsiveness of the visual cortex to visual stimulation. This additional data helps determine the degree of functional impairment and inform treatment decisions. The precision MRI and fMRI provide assists in distinguishing between different types of optic neuropathies, differentiating between inflammatory and ischemic causes, and helping guide treatment tailored to the specific pathology.

The advantages of utilizing both MRI and fMRI extend beyond specific diagnoses. These techniques provide valuable insights into the intricate workings of the visual system. Studies employing fMRI have mapped the neural pathways involved in various visual tasks, clarifying how the brain processes different visual stimuli. This fundamental research significantly informs our understanding of visual perception, contributing to a broader understanding of visual processing mechanisms and potential deficits. For example, researchers can study how different visual stimuli activate various parts of the brain, and this enhanced understanding informs our treatments. Understanding the functional connectivity between different brain regions involved in visual processing can potentially lead to novel therapeutic interventions.

It's also important to remember that interpretation of MRI and fMRI data requires expertise. Radiologists and neuro-ophthalmologists must work together, correlating imaging findings with clinical presentation and other diagnostic tests. The images themselves are only part of the diagnostic process, and thorough clinical assessment is indispensable for accurate diagnosis and management. The interpretation of any abnormal findings must always be taken in the context of the patient's overall clinical picture. The power of MRI and fMRI lies in their ability to provide detailed information; however, clinical correlation is paramount for accurate interpretation.

Finally, advancements in MRI and fMRI technology continue to improve the resolution and sensitivity of these techniques. Newer sequences offer enhanced visualization of subtle lesions and improved detection of functional changes. The ongoing development of sophisticated image analysis software facilitates more quantitative and objective assessment of imaging data. Future research will likely focus on developing even more sophisticated techniques for studying the visual system, helping refine diagnoses and improve patient outcomes. Therefore, staying abreast of technological advancements will be crucial for practitioners in this field.

## 4.3 Visual Evoked Potentials

Visual evoked potentials (VEPs) are invaluable tools in neuro-ophthalmology, providing a non-invasive window into the functional integrity of the visual pathways. They measure the electrical activity in the brain elicited by visual stimulation, revealing the time course and amplitude of neural responses along different stages of visual processing. This information is crucial for diagnosing and monitoring various neurological conditions affecting vision.

Unlike structural imaging techniques such as MRI or OCT that primarily show anatomical details, VEPs offer a dynamic assessment of how the visual system responds to stimuli. The test is relatively simple to administer, requiring the patient to look at a pattern-reversal checkerboard or other visual stimuli while electrodes on the scalp record the brain's electrical responses. These responses, which are typically small, are then amplified and analyzed.

The latency and amplitude of different VEP components provide valuable insights. For instance, prolonged latency can indicate slowed nerve conduction, suggestive of demyelination as seen in multiple sclerosis or optic neuritis. Reduced amplitude, on the other hand, may point towards damage or dysfunction along the visual pathway. Different components of the VEP reflect activity at different stages of the pathway, from the retina to the visual cortex. Therefore, analyzing the various components allows for a more precise localization of the lesion.

Pattern-reversal VEPs are commonly used to assess the function of the optic nerves, optic tracts, and visual cortex. Flash VEPs, using a bright flash of light as a stimulus, are often employed to evaluate more broadly the integrity of the retina and optic nerve. Each type of VEP offers unique diagnostic advantages depending on the specific clinical question and suspected pathology. Careful consideration of the appropriate VEP type is paramount for achieving accurate results.

The interpretation of VEPs requires expertise in both electrophysiology and neuro-ophthalmology. A skilled clinician will analyze the waveforms, considering factors such as age, refractive error, and overall patient health. Furthermore, the VEP results should always be interpreted in conjunction with other clinical findings, such as visual acuity, visual field testing, and imaging studies. A comprehensive approach is essential for a correct diagnosis.

While VEPs are a powerful diagnostic tool, they do have limitations. They are not always able to precisely pinpoint the exact location of a lesion, especially small or subtle lesions. False-positive and false-negative results are possible, influenced by factors like patient cooperation and technical artifacts. Moreover, VEPs may be abnormal in individuals without clinically apparent visual dysfunction, emphasizing the importance of a holistic assessment.

Despite these limitations, VEPs remain an invaluable diagnostic and monitoring tool in neuro-ophthalmology. Their non-invasive nature makes them particularly suitable for repeated examinations over time, allowing clinicians to monitor disease progression or treatment response in conditions such as multiple sclerosis or optic neuritis. By offering a window into the functional integrity of the visual system, VEPs contribute significantly to the comprehensive care of patients with neuro-ophthalmological conditions. The information gained from VEPs complements findings from other investigations and aids in refining diagnostic accuracy and guiding treatment decisions, ultimately improving patient outcomes. Understanding the application and interpretation of VEPs is an essential skill for any neuro-ophthalmologist. Integrating these results with other clinical findings is critical in reaching informed, precise diagnoses. In conjunction with other diagnostic tools, VEPs offer an advanced understanding of visual pathway functionality that isn't obtainable otherwise.

# 5 Neurological Basis of Visual Disorders

Understanding the neurological basis of visual disorders requires a grasp of how the brain processes visual information. The intricate network connecting the eyes to the visual cortex is vulnerable to various pathologies, leading to a range of visual impairments. Consider, for instance, the disruption of signals at the optic chiasm, a crucial point where fibers from each eye cross. Damage here can create specific visual field deficits, such as bitemporal hemianopia, where vision is lost in the outer halves of both visual fields. This illustrates the direct link between neurological compromise and observable visual dysfunction.
Diplopia, or double vision, frequently stems from disruptions in the coordination of eye movements. The extraocular muscles, controlled by cranial nerves III, IV, and VI, precisely regulate eye alignment. Neurological conditions affecting these nerves, such as a stroke or aneurysm, or damage to their nuclei in the brainstem can impair this control, resulting in misaligned eyes and the perception of two images. Precise diagnosis requires detailed neuro-ophthalmological examination, identifying the affected nerve or muscle and the nature of the neurological insult. This underlines the crucial role of a collaborative approach involving both ophthalmologists and neurologists.
Visual field defects manifest in numerous ways, providing valuable clues to the location and nature of the neurological lesion. A lesion in the optic nerve, for example, will cause monocular vision loss, affecting only one eye. Conversely, a lesion in the optic tract, after the optic

chiasm, results in a homonymous hemianopia, affecting the same half of the visual field in both eyes. More complex defects, such as quadrantanopias (loss of a quarter of the visual field) or macular sparing (preservation of central vision), further refine localization of the lesion within the visual pathways. Careful mapping of the visual field defect is paramount for accurate diagnosis and guiding neuroimaging investigations. Careful clinical observation becomes an invaluable diagnostic tool.

Color vision deficits offer another facet in the diagnostic puzzle. The ability to discriminate colors is primarily determined by the activity of three types of cone photoreceptors within the retina, each sensitive to different wavelengths of light. Neurological lesions affecting the central visual pathways, particularly the V4 area of the visual cortex, responsible for color perception, can cause acquired color vision deficiencies. These are distinct from congenital color blindness, which has a genetic origin. Assessment often involves standardized color vision tests, such as the Ishihara plates, to pinpoint the nature and extent of the color vision impairment. The diagnostic significance of these deficits lies in the fact that they are quite specific to certain types of lesions.

Strabismus, characterized by misalignment of the eyes, can have both neurological and non-neurological causes. While refractive errors and other ocular factors can contribute, neurological conditions, such as cerebral palsy or tumors affecting the brainstem or cranial nerves, can also lead to strabismus. The specific type of strabismus (esotropia, exotropia, hypertropia, hypotropia) helps pinpoint the underlying neurological abnormality. Diagnosis often requires a comprehensive assessment combining ophthalmological examination with neurological evaluation and neuroimaging. The interaction between eye muscle imbalances and neurological causes underscores the interdisciplinary nature of neuro-ophthalmology.

In essence, understanding the neurological basis of visual disorders necessitates an appreciation of the intricate interplay between the visual system's anatomical structures and their neurological control. Each visual disorder discussed—diplopia, visual field defects, color vision deficiencies, and strabismus—reveals crucial insights into the brain's visual processing mechanisms and its vulnerability to various neurological insults. A detailed neuro-ophthalmological examination, utilizing advanced neuroimaging techniques, is essential for accurate diagnosis and guiding effective management strategies. This diagnostic process allows us to uncover the intricate connections between the neurological and visual aspects of the patient's condition.

## 5.1 Diplopia and Strabismus

Double vision, or diplopia, and strabismus, a misalignment of the eyes, are common neuro-ophthalmological conditions impacting visual perception and eye coordination. Understanding their underlying neurological mechanisms is crucial for effective diagnosis and management.
Diplopia arises when the brain fails to fuse the slightly different images received from each eye, leading to the perception of two superimposed images. This can stem from various causes, including cranial nerve palsies affecting the extraocular muscles responsible for eye movement, neuromuscular junction disorders impacting muscle function, or lesions affecting the brainstem nuclei that control these muscles. Accurate diagnosis necessitates a thorough neurological examination, focusing on cranial nerve function and eye muscle strength.
Strabismus, conversely, represents a deviation in the visual axis of one or both eyes. It can be congenital, present from birth due to developmental abnormalities, or acquired, resulting from neurological conditions, such as stroke or trauma. Esotropia, where the eye turns inward, and exotropia, where the eye turns outward, are common types. The neurological underpinnings involve imbalances in the innervation and control of the extraocular muscles, often due to dysfunction within the brainstem's oculomotor centers or the pathways connecting them to the muscles themselves. Imaging techniques, such as magnetic resonance imaging (MRI), can be invaluable in identifying underlying structural lesions responsible for acquired strabismus.
The clinical presentation of diplopia and strabismus varies depend-

ing on their etiology and severity. In diplopia, the patient experiences double vision, often described as seeing two overlapping images. The discomfort can be significant, particularly when attempting visually demanding tasks. Strabismus manifests as a visible misalignment of the eyes, potentially causing amblyopia ("lazy eye") in children if left untreated, as one eye's image is suppressed to avoid double vision. Careful observation of eye movements and pupillary reflexes during a comprehensive ophthalmological and neurological examination is vital for assessment.

Treatment strategies for diplopia and strabismus are tailored to the underlying cause. If a cranial nerve palsy is identified, treatment might focus on addressing the underlying neurological condition. For example, corticosteroid therapy may be used to manage inflammation related to nerve compression. In cases of myasthenia gravis, affecting neuromuscular transmission, acetylcholinesterase inhibitors might improve muscle function. Surgical intervention may be necessary to correct muscle imbalances causing strabismus. Precise surgical adjustments of the extraocular muscles can restore proper alignment and improve binocular vision.

Rehabilitative therapies play a significant role in the management of both diplopia and strabismus, particularly in cases where complete cure isn't feasible. Orthoptic exercises, designed to improve eye coordination and binocular fusion, can be highly beneficial. These exercises often involve training the eyes to work together, focusing on convergence and divergence, thus reducing the perception of double vision and improving eye alignment. In children with strabismus, patching the stronger eye can stimulate the weaker eye's development, helping to prevent or correct amblyopia. These therapies require patience and commitment from the patient.

Advanced imaging techniques, such as MRI and functional MRI (fMRI), are increasingly important in the diagnosis of diplopia and strabismus. MRI allows the visualization of brain structures, helping to identify tumors, strokes, or other lesions that might cause cranial nerve palsies or affect brainstem oculomotor centers. fMRI can assess the functional activity of the visual pathways and oculomotor control regions, providing insights into the neural mechanisms underlying these conditions. These tools, combined with detailed neurological examination, enable a comprehensive evaluation of the patient's condition.

The prognosis for diplopia and strabismus varies greatly based on etiology and the response to treatment. In some cases, complete resolution of symptoms is achievable, especially with early intervention and appropriate management. For example, successful treatment of an underlying neurological condition often leads to the recovery of normal binocular vision. Other cases might require ongoing management, with regular orthoptic exercises and possibly further surgical interventions. It's crucial to manage expectations, tailoring communication about potential outcomes to the individual situation. A multidisciplinary approach, involving neurologists, ophthalmologists, and orthoptists, often provides the best results. Ongoing research explores novel therapeutic strategies to improve outcomes in these conditions, emphasizing the importance of interdisciplinary collaboration.

Understanding the intricate interplay between neurological function and visual perception is vital in neuro-ophthalmology. Diplopia and strabismus, though seemingly simple visual problems, highlight the complex neural mechanisms governing eye movements and binocular vision. Accurate diagnosis, based on a thorough clinical assessment and appropriate imaging studies, combined with tailored treatment strategies – encompassing medical, surgical, and rehabilitative approaches – is key to achieving optimal visual outcomes and improving the quality of life for affected individuals. The advancements in neuroimaging and our growing understanding of the neurological control of eye movements continue to improve both diagnosis and therapy, emphasizing the interconnectedness of neurology and ophthalmology in managing these conditions. Furthermore, the integration of advanced imaging techniques within this framework allows for more precise diagnoses and treatment plans, improving patient outcomes. Early identification and intervention, therefore, remain critical to achieving the best possible results.

## 5.2 Visual Field Defects

Understanding visual field defects requires a grasp of the visual pathway's intricate architecture. Imagine the pathway as a complex network of roads carrying visual information from the eyes to the brain's visual processing center. Damage at any point along this route can disrupt the flow, leading to characteristic visual field loss. This loss isn't random; it's highly predictable, reflecting the specific location and extent of the lesion.

A common pattern is a homonymous hemianopia. This means loss of vision in the same half of the visual field in both eyes. For instance, someone might lose their entire right visual field in both eyes, a classic sign of damage affecting the optic tract or visual cortex on the left side of the brain. The brain's organization ensures that each eye's visual field contributes to a single visual image.

Consider the impact of a lesion affecting the optic nerve. This would result in unilateral visual loss, affecting one eye entirely. A lesion near the optic chiasm, where the optic nerves cross, can create a distinctive bitemporal hemianopia—loss of the temporal (outer) visual fields in both eyes. This occurs because the nasal (inner) fibers from each eye, carrying information from the temporal visual field, cross at the chiasm. Damage here interrupts this crossing information.

Lesions further down the pathway, within the optic radiations or the visual cortex itself, can produce more complex patterns of visual field loss, often affecting specific quadrants or sectors of the visual field. The precise location of the damage dictates the specific nature of the defect. For example, damage to the inferior optic radiations typically causes a superior quadrantanopia – loss of vision in the upper half of the visual field in one or both eyes.

Precise localization of these lesions is paramount. Careful history-taking, coupled with thorough visual field testing, is critical. Perimetry, a standardized method for mapping the visual field, is a cornerstone of this assessment. This involves systematically presenting visual stimuli at various locations within the visual field and recording the patient's responses. The resulting map reveals areas of visual loss and their precise boundaries.

However, perimetry alone isn't sufficient for complete diagnosis. It's crucial to integrate these findings with neuroimaging techniques, such as MRI or CT scans, to pinpoint the lesion's location and size. Neuroimaging can reveal structural abnormalities, such as tumors, infarcts, or demyelinating lesions, providing a crucial piece of the diagnostic puzzle.

The specific treatment strategy will depend on the underlying cause of the visual field defect. For example, if a tumor is responsible, surgical intervention or radiation therapy might be necessary. If an ischemic event caused the loss, aggressive management of risk factors and sometimes medication to prevent further events will be the focus. In cases of demyelination, medications modulating the immune system might be used.

In some cases, despite the best medical management, the visual field defect may persist. In such scenarios, rehabilitation and adaptive strategies become crucial. Low vision aids, such as magnifiers or specialized software, can help individuals compensate for their visual loss and maintain independence in daily life. Occupational therapy can assist in adapting daily routines, enhancing the efficiency of remaining visual function.

The prognosis varies significantly depending on the underlying pathology and the extent of the visual field defect. While some conditions, such as those caused by minor strokes, might lead to some recovery, others, especially those with major causes or long duration, may leave lasting visual impairments. Early detection and swift intervention are critical for maximizing the chance of a favorable outcome, improving visual function and quality of life. In the context of neuro-ophthalmology, a multidisciplinary approach involving ophthalmologists, neurologists, and rehabilitation specialists is most effective in providing optimal care for patients with visual field defects. The journey towards accurate diagnosis and effective management often requires this collaborative approach. It emphasizes the interconnectedness of neurological and ophthalmological systems and the vital importance of understanding their interaction in addressing a wide range of conditions affecting vision.

## 5.3 Color Vision Deficits

Understanding color vision relies on specialized cone photoreceptor cells within the retina, each sensitive to different wavelengths of light – red, green, and blue. These cones, working in concert, send signals along the optic nerve, ultimately processed in the visual cortex to create our perception of color. Disruptions anywhere along this pathway can lead to color vision deficits, also known as color blindness.

The most common cause is genetic, often inherited in an X-linked recessive manner. This means that men are disproportionately affected, as they only possess one X chromosome. Women, having two X chromosomes, usually need two affected genes to manifest the condition, making it less prevalent in the female population. These genetic defects typically affect the production or function of one or more cone types, resulting in difficulty distinguishing specific colors.

Red-green color blindness is the most frequently observed type. Individuals might struggle to differentiate between shades of red and green, leading to challenges in everyday activities, such as traffic signal recognition or picking ripe fruits. Blue-yellow color blindness, while less common, presents similar difficulties with distinguishing colors within those spectral ranges. Complete color blindness, or achromatopsia, is rare and characterized by a lack of color perception, resulting in a world seen only in shades of gray.

Beyond genetics, acquired color vision deficits can arise from various neurological conditions. Damage to the optic nerve, the pathway carrying visual signals from the eye to the brain, can impair color perception. Conditions like optic neuritis, an inflammation of the optic nerve, or glaucoma, characterized by increased intraocular pressure damaging the optic nerve, are prime examples. Lesions within the visual cortex, the brain area responsible for visual processing, can also disrupt color vision, leading to deficits that may vary widely depending on the location and extent of the damage.

Diagnosing color vision deficits involves a range of tests. The Ishihara plates, a series of colored dots arranged to form numbers, are a common and widely accessible screening tool. These tests identify individuals with difficulties perceiving specific color combinations. More detailed assessments utilize anomaloscopes, instruments that allow for precise measurement of color matching abilities, providing a more quantitative evaluation of the extent of the deficit. These specialized tools assist in characterizing the exact nature of the color vision deficiency.

Treatment approaches for color vision deficits predominantly focus on compensatory strategies rather than curing the underlying condition. For inherited color blindness, there's no current cure. However, the use of color-correcting lenses or filters can help improve color discrimination in some individuals. These aids filter out certain wavelengths of light, effectively improving the contrast between colors that are difficult to distinguish otherwise.

In cases of acquired color vision deficits stemming from neurological conditions, addressing the underlying cause is crucial. Treating conditions like optic neuritis or glaucoma can potentially improve or stabilize color vision. However, recovery depends significantly on the severity and location of the damage, as well as the time elapsed since the onset of the condition. For example, prompt treatment of optic neuritis can be essential to preserve visual function, including color vision. In cases of significant irreversible damage, rehabilitative therapies and assistive technologies may play a vital role in helping individuals adapt and function effectively in their daily lives. This involves learning coping mechanisms and adapting to the challenges posed by impaired color vision.

For professionals working with individuals experiencing color vision deficits, understanding the variety of potential causes and appropriate diagnostic methods is essential. This understanding enables them to offer informed advice and guide individuals toward appropriate support and adaptive strategies. Emphasizing that many everyday tasks can be accommodated with practical adjustments significantly improves their quality of life. It is crucial to approach this topic with sensitivity and practicality, focusing on strategies that enable individuals to maintain their independence and self-reliance.

# 6 Therapeutic Interventions

Effective treatment in neuro-ophthalmology hinges on a multi-pronged approach, combining medication, surgery, and rehabilitation. The specific intervention will depend heavily on the underlying condition and its severity, always tailored to the individual patient's needs and response. Careful consideration of each patient's unique circumstances is crucial for optimal results.

Medical management forms the cornerstone of therapy for many neuro-ophthalmological conditions. For example, in optic neuritis, high-dose corticosteroids are frequently administered to reduce inflammation and expedite recovery, potentially lessening the impact on visual acuity. Intravenous methylprednisolone is often the first choice, followed by oral prednisone tapering. In cases of ischemic optic neuropathy, while there's no definitive cure, supportive measures such as blood pressure control and management of underlying vascular conditions are paramount. Some patients may benefit from medications to improve blood flow. Close monitoring is essential throughout the treatment period. The choice of medication and dosage should always align with the specific diagnosis and the patient's overall health profile. Beyond corticosteroids, other medications, like immunomodulators, may be used depending on the diagnosis and individual responses.

Surgical intervention plays a significant role in selected cases. For example, strabismus, a condition resulting in misalignment of the eyes, often necessitates surgical correction to realign the extraocular muscles and improve binocular vision. This procedure aims to restore proper muscle balance for improved eye coordination and reduced double vision. Precise surgical techniques, informed by pre-operative assessments, are crucial for achieving the desired outcome, minimizing potential complications, and ensuring the patient's overall comfort. Advanced imaging techniques, including high-resolution MRI, are invaluable in planning surgical approaches and reducing potential complications. The choice to proceed with surgery involves careful consideration of the benefits and risks against the patient's specific circumstances and health condition.

Rehabilitative therapies offer a complementary approach to managing visual impairments arising from neuro-ophthalmological disorders. Vision therapy, for instance, is a personalized program of exercises designed to enhance visual skills such as eye coordination, visual acuity, and visual fields. It involves specialized exercises, often guided by an optometrist or orthoptist, to improve eye muscle function, focusing ability, and visual perception. It is often paired with other visual therapies to optimize the rehabilitation process. Low vision rehabilitation, tailored to patients with significant visual impairments, focuses on adaptive strategies to maximize functional vision in everyday life. This might include the use of assistive devices like magnifying glasses or special lighting, strategies for improved reading or mobility, and training in daily living skills. Furthermore, occupational therapy plays a significant role in adapting the patient's surroundings and routines to help compensate for vision difficulties. The therapist will assess the needs and identify areas needing assistance or adaptation.

The prognosis for neuro-ophthalmological conditions varies widely depending on the underlying pathology, the stage at which intervention begins, and the individual patient's response to treatment. Early diagnosis and prompt intervention are typically associated with more favorable outcomes, particularly in conditions like optic neuritis. However, even with timely treatment, some visual impairments may persist. In these instances, the focus shifts towards managing existing deficits and enhancing the patient's quality of life through rehabilitative therapies. Continuous monitoring and follow-up are crucial for managing complications, adjusting treatment plans as needed, and optimizing the patient's visual function and well-being.

Ultimately, a collaborative approach involving neurologists, ophthalmologists, optometrists, and rehabilitation specialists is essential for delivering optimal care. This team-based approach allows for comprehensive evaluation, tailored treatment planning, and coordinated management throughout the patient's journey. Open communication among healthcare professionals and the patient ensures informed decision-making and promotes active participation in the treatment process. The overarching goal is to improve visual function, enhance quality of life, and support the patient's successful adaptation to any persisting visual challenges.

## 6.1 Medical Management Strategies

Effective medical management in neuro-ophthalmology hinges on a precise diagnosis, followed by a tailored treatment plan that addresses the underlying cause of the visual dysfunction. This often involves a multidisciplinary approach, drawing upon the expertise of neurologists, ophthalmologists, and other specialists as needed. The specific strategies employed will vary depending on the condition, its severity, and the patient's overall health.

Early intervention is paramount in many neuro-ophthalmological disorders. Delaying treatment can lead to irreversible vision loss, emphasizing the importance of prompt diagnosis and initiation of therapy. For example, in acute optic neuritis, corticosteroids can help reduce inflammation and potentially prevent permanent visual impairment, but their efficacy is significantly higher when administered promptly.

Pharmacological interventions often form the cornerstone of medical management. Corticosteroids, like methylprednisolone, are frequently used to combat inflammation in conditions such as optic neuritis and uveitis. Other medications might target specific underlying causes, such as autoimmune diseases or infections. The choice of medication, dosage, and duration of treatment are carefully considered based on the individual patient's needs and response to therapy. Regular monitoring of visual acuity, visual fields, and other relevant parameters is crucial to assess treatment efficacy and adjust the treatment plan as necessary.

Beyond corticosteroids, other medications play vital roles. For example, immunomodulatory agents may be necessary in cases of autoimmune-mediated optic neuropathies. These medications help to suppress the immune system's attack on the optic nerve. Careful monitoring is crucial to avoid potential side effects and ensure the treatment's effectiveness. The goal isn't just to stop the progression of the disease but to improve visual function where possible.

Nutritional support can play a surprisingly important role in certain cases. A balanced diet rich in antioxidants and vitamins may help to protect the visual system from damage and promote healing. However, this is considered a supportive measure rather than a primary treatment and should always be discussed with a healthcare professional. Specific dietary recommendations will depend on the individual patient's condition and overall health status.

Regular follow-up appointments are essential for ongoing monitoring and assessment. This allows for early detection of any complications or changes in the patient's condition, ensuring prompt adjustments to the treatment plan. Consistent monitoring is particularly important with conditions that can progress subtly over time, such as glaucoma. These appointments also provide a forum for the patient to express any concerns and receive tailored advice on managing their condition. This collaborative approach between the patient and the healthcare team is crucial for success.

Furthermore, patient education is vital. Understanding their condition, treatment plan, and potential side effects empowers patients to actively participate in their care. This can lead to improved adherence to the treatment regimen and better overall outcomes. Clear and accessible communication, coupled with written materials and support groups, can enhance patient understanding and reduce anxiety.

In summary, effective medical management in neuro-ophthalmology demands a holistic, personalized approach. It involves a careful assessment of the individual patient's condition, a timely and targeted treatment strategy that integrates pharmacological interventions, nutritional support, and ongoing monitoring. Regular follow-up appointments and patient education are crucial to ensure optimal outcomes and improve the patient's quality of life. The ultimate goal is not only to treat the immediate symptoms but to protect vision and prevent further deterioration. The complexity of neuro-ophthalmological conditions often necessitates a coordinated team of specialists working together to achieve the best possible results for the patient. Through close collaboration and careful management, significant improvements in visual function and overall well-being are attainable. The emphasis should always remain on providing compassionate and comprehensive care to optimize the patient's quality of life.

## 6.2 Surgical Options

Surgical intervention in neuro-ophthalmology is often a last resort, employed when medical management fails to provide adequate improvement or when the underlying condition necessitates direct surgical intervention. Consider the case of a patient with severe compressive optic neuropathy due to an orbital tumor. Medical treatment might involve steroids to reduce inflammation, but if the tumor continues to grow, causing irreversible vision loss, surgery becomes necessary to remove the mass and alleviate pressure on the optic nerve. The timing of such interventions is critical, balancing the urgency of the situation with the potential risks of surgery.
The specific surgical procedures utilized depend entirely on the underlying cause of the neurological visual impairment. For example, decompression surgeries are common in cases of compressive lesions, such as those caused by orbital tumors or aneurysms. These procedures aim to relieve pressure on the optic nerve or other structures of the visual pathway. The approach can vary, depending on the location and nature of the compression. Sometimes a minimally invasive procedure may suffice; other times, a more extensive cranial or orbital surgery is required. Postoperative management often includes close monitoring of visual function and management of any complications.

In cases of strabismus, surgery focuses on realigning the eyes to improve binocular vision. This typically involves adjusting the extraocular muscles, which control eye movement. Precise measurements and surgical planning are crucial to achieve optimal alignment, while minimizing the risk of complications such as double vision or eye movement restrictions. Postoperative rehabilitation often involves patching or the use of prisms to help the brain adapt to the new alignment. Success rates are high, but individual outcomes depend on factors like the patient's age and the severity of the strabismus.

Certain lesions of the optic nerve may be amenable to surgical intervention, such as optic nerve sheath fenestration, which involves creating a small opening in the sheath surrounding the optic nerve to relieve pressure from cerebrospinal fluid buildup. This procedure is particularly relevant in cases of papilledema, where increased intracranial pressure leads to swelling of the optic disc. Careful patient selection and surgical technique are essential to minimize the risk of complications such as bleeding or further damage to the optic nerve. The long-term success often depends on managing the underlying cause of the increased intracranial pressure.

Surgical management of aneurysms affecting the visual pathways presents unique challenges due to their location in the brain or orbit. Microsurgical techniques, often employing advanced imaging guidance, allow neurosurgeons to carefully clip or coil the aneurysm, preventing further bleeding and damage to the visual pathways. Postoperative recovery can be lengthy and requires meticulous monitoring for any signs of recurrence or other complications. The expertise of both neurosurgeons and neuro-ophthalmologists is often crucial in this type of complex surgery.

Ultimately, the decision to proceed with surgical intervention is based on a careful consideration of several factors. The severity of the visual impairment, the responsiveness to medical therapies, the presence of comorbidities and the associated surgical risks must all be thoroughly evaluated before proceeding. The neuro-ophthalmologist plays a critical role in this decision-making process. They work collaboratively with other specialists, such as neurosurgeons and ophthalmologists, to create the best individualized treatment strategy. This multidisciplinary approach ensures the best possible outcome for the patient while minimizing potential risks. Therefore, a collaborative and comprehensive approach is imperative for optimal surgical outcomes in neuro-ophthalmology. This ensures the patient receives the most appropriate and effective care.

## 6.3 Rehabilitative Therapies

Rehabilitative therapies play a crucial role in improving visual function and quality of life for individuals affected by neuro-ophthalmological conditions. These therapies are not merely supplementary; they are often integral to achieving the best possible visual outcomes, particularly after conditions like optic neuritis or stroke affecting the visual pathways.

Many rehabilitation strategies aim to enhance the brain's plasticity, its remarkable ability to reorganize itself after injury or disease. This adaptive capacity enables the brain to compensate for damaged areas by recruiting other neural networks. Techniques such as visual field exercises and perceptual learning capitalize on this plasticity.

Visual field exercises, for example, might involve targeted practice using specialized computer programs or vision therapy games. These programs carefully present visual stimuli within the affected visual field, gradually expanding the area of awareness and improving sensitivity. The goal is to stimulate the brain's residual visual pathways, encouraging them to become more active and responsive. Regular, consistent practice is key to seeing meaningful improvement.

Perceptual learning, another powerful rehabilitative tool, focuses on training the brain to interpret and process visual information more effectively. This may involve repeated tasks like identifying shapes, colors, or patterns in cluttered backgrounds. This method helps the brain to compensate for deficits in processing speed or visual acuity by improving visual perception and attention. Practitioners often adjust the difficulty of exercises to optimize the patient's engagement and progress.

Beyond specialized exercises, compensatory strategies can greatly enhance daily life. These involve adapting to visual field deficits through changes in behavior and environment. For someone with hemianopsia (loss of half the visual field), for instance, systematic head turning or using scanning techniques to cover the entire visual field can greatly improve functional vision. Environmental modifications, such as strategically placing objects within the preserved visual field or using assistive devices like prism glasses, can also prove invaluable.

Low vision aids also hold significant potential. These devices include magnifiers, large-print materials, and electronic visual aids that enhance contrast or enlarge images. Careful selection of low vision aids must consider the individual's specific visual impairment and lifestyle needs, maximizing their effectiveness. A comprehensive low vision assessment conducted by a certified low vision therapist is crucial in this process.

Beyond the practical strategies, emotional support and counseling form a vital component of comprehensive rehabilitation. Neuro-ophthalmological conditions can significantly impact a patient's self-esteem, independence, and mental well-being. The psychological effects of visual impairment should not be overlooked, and therapeutic interventions should address the patient's emotional needs. Support groups or individual counseling can provide much needed encouragement and coping strategies, improving overall adjustment and compliance with treatment. This is often crucial for successful long-term rehabilitation.

Furthermore, the rehabilitation process is highly individualized, and requires a collaborative approach. Regular monitoring of progress is essential. Progress is not always linear. There may be plateaus, periods of improvement followed by apparent setbacks. Close collaboration among ophthalmologists, neurologists, low vision therapists, and occupational therapists allows for ongoing adjustment of therapy based on the individual's specific responses, and ensures the therapy remains focused and effective. This interdisciplinary approach is crucial for achieving optimal visual outcomes.

The integration of technology also offers exciting opportunities in rehabilitative therapies. Virtual reality (VR) systems, for example, can provide immersive environments for training visual skills, making the therapy more engaging and motivating. VR allows the creation of tailored scenarios that mimic real-life situations, thus promoting better generalization of learned skills to everyday activities. As VR technology evolves, its applications in neuro-ophthalmological rehabilitation will likely increase significantly. This could provide personalized and highly effective approaches for a wide range of visual impairments. Early adoption of such technologies is warranted, given the immense potential they hold for patient recovery and improved quality of life.

# 7 Future Directions in Neuro-Ophthalmology

The integration of artificial intelligence and machine learning holds immense potential for revolutionizing diagnostic accuracy. Imagine a system capable of analyzing retinal scans with unparalleled precision, identifying subtle indicators of neurological damage invisible to the human eye. This level of automated analysis could lead to earlier diagnoses and more targeted interventions, ultimately improving patient outcomes. Furthermore, AI-driven predictive models could forecast disease progression, enabling proactive management strategies and potentially delaying or even preventing significant vision loss. Developing advanced gene therapies represents a significant frontier. Currently, several research groups are actively investigating gene-editing techniques to address the genetic underpinnings of inherited neuro-ophthalmological conditions. This groundbreaking work could potentially offer curative treatments for previously untreatable diseases, transforming the lives of countless individuals and their families. However, substantial research and rigorous clinical trials are necessary to ensure safety and efficacy before widespread implementation.

Neuro-imaging techniques continue to evolve at a rapid pace. Higher-resolution MRI and fMRI scanners are constantly being developed, providing ever-finer detail of the visual pathways. This improved resolution allows for more precise localization of lesions, better characterization of disease processes, and improved monitoring of treatment response. Furthermore, advanced image analysis techniques, leveraging AI and machine learning, can enhance the interpretation of neuroimaging data, making the diagnostic process faster and more efficient. Beyond imaging, innovative neuro-protective agents are actively being explored. These agents aim to enhance the resilience of neural tissues, mitigating damage from ischemia, inflammation, or trauma. Preclinical studies using animal models are yielding promising results, suggesting that these neuroprotective therapies could offer significant therapeutic benefits in the future. The translation of these preclinical successes into effective human therapies is, however, a challenging but crucial next step.

The field of personalized medicine is poised to transform neuro-ophthalmological care. As our understanding of the genetic and environmental factors that contribute to neuro-ophthalmological diseases grows, we can begin to tailor treatment plans to individual patients based on their unique profiles. This approach, combining genetic testing with advanced imaging and clinical data, can significantly enhance treatment efficacy and minimize adverse effects. This move toward personalized approaches necessitates more investment in large-scale genomic studies, linking specific genetic variations to disease phenotypes.

Collaborative research efforts are increasingly important. The complexity of the visual system requires interdisciplinary collaboration, bringing together ophthalmologists, neurologists, geneticists, computer scientists, and engineers. Joint research endeavors will be vital for unlocking the full potential of emerging technologies and accelerating the development of novel diagnostic and therapeutic tools. This concerted effort needs to be supported by increased funding for research, fostering an environment where diverse teams can collaborate effectively.

The development of novel rehabilitative therapies shows great promise. Current rehabilitative techniques focus primarily on adapting to visual deficits, but future therapies might aim at actively repairing damaged neural circuits. This could involve advanced sensory stimulation techniques, pharmacological interventions, or even direct neural stimulation to improve visual function. This exciting area requires a multifaceted approach, combining innovative therapeutic strategies with rigorous clinical evaluations.

Improved access to care remains a critical issue. Many individuals with neuro-ophthalmological conditions lack access to timely and appropriate care, particularly in resource-limited settings. Telemedicine offers a promising solution, enabling remote diagnosis and monitoring of patients, regardless of geographical location. However, ensuring equitable access to telemedicine platforms and supporting infrastructure is essential to bridging the gap in healthcare access globally. The need for training healthcare professionals in this area is paramount for successful implementation.

In conclusion, the future of neuro-ophthalmology is bright. The convergence of emerging technologies, innovative therapies, and collaborative research initiatives will significantly advance our understanding and treatment of neuro-ophthalmological conditions. Overcoming the remaining challenges, particularly in terms of gene therapy translation and ensuring equitable access to advanced technologies, will be critical in achieving our ultimate goal: dramatically improving the lives of those affected by these debilitating conditions. Continuous refinement of imaging techniques and the expansion of AI applications will be pivotal steps toward more precise diagnoses and more effective therapeutic interventions.

## 7.1 Emerging Technologies

Optical coherence tomography (OCT) angiography, a non-invasive imaging modality, offers a significant leap forward in visualizing the retinal and choroidal vasculature. Its ability to detect subtle changes in blood flow, previously undetectable with conventional OCT, promises earlier diagnosis and monitoring of conditions like age-related macular degeneration and diabetic retinopathy, both often associated with neurological involvement. This improved visualization allows for a more precise understanding of disease progression and the effectiveness of therapeutic interventions. The detailed vascular maps generated by OCT angiography are invaluable for neuro-ophthalmologists, providing crucial insights into the relationship between vascular health and neurological function within the visual system. The non-invasive nature minimizes patient discomfort, enhancing the diagnostic process.

Artificial intelligence (AI) algorithms are being increasingly integrated into image analysis software for neuro-ophthalmological imaging. These algorithms can automate the detection of subtle abnormalities that might be missed by the human eye, improving diagnostic accuracy and efficiency. For instance, AI can analyze OCT scans to identify early signs of glaucomatous damage to the optic nerve, potentially leading to earlier intervention and preventing irreversible vision loss. Similarly, AI can assist in the interpretation of visual field tests, helping to identify patterns indicative of specific neurological conditions impacting vision. This technology promises to significantly reduce diagnostic error rates and improve the efficiency of neuro-ophthalmological practices, ultimately benefiting a greater number of patients.

Beyond image analysis, AI also holds the potential for personalized medicine in neuro-ophthalmology. By analyzing large datasets of patient information—including imaging data, clinical notes, and genetic information—AI algorithms can identify patterns and predict individual patient responses to different treatment options. This capability could lead to more tailored and effective therapeutic strategies, optimizing visual outcomes and improving the overall quality of life for patients with neuro-ophthalmological conditions. This personalized approach could particularly benefit patients with complex conditions requiring individualized treatment plans. Moreover, ongoing research explores the potential of AI to predict disease progression, allowing for proactive interventions.

Advancements in gene therapy show tremendous promise for treating various neuro-ophthalmological diseases. Researchers are exploring targeted gene delivery systems to correct genetic defects that cause conditions like retinitis pigmentosa, a degenerative eye disease affecting photoreceptor cells and often linked to neurological impairments.

Gene therapy approaches aim to either replace defective genes or introduce new genes to restore or enhance the function of damaged cells. While still in its early stages for many neuro-ophthalmological applications, the successes observed in other fields suggest significant potential for improving visual outcomes and quality of life for patients affected by inherited visual disorders that have a strong correlation with neurological function. Clinical trials are underway to evaluate the safety and efficacy of different gene therapy strategies for a range of conditions.

Brain-computer interfaces (BCIs) are emerging as a potential therapeutic approach for patients with severe visual impairment due to neurological conditions. BCIs work by translating neural signals from the brain into commands that can control external devices, such as prosthetic eyes or visual display systems. For those with irreversible damage to the visual pathways, BCIs offer a completely novel pathway to restore some level of vision. These systems are becoming increasingly sophisticated, allowing for greater levels of precision and control. While still in their developmental stages, BCIs represent a radical shift in the treatment paradigm for severe visual loss, providing hope for patients previously considered untreatable. The potential to bypass damaged parts of the visual pathway using brain signals opens entirely new avenues of rehabilitation.

High-resolution functional magnetic resonance imaging (fMRI) and other neuroimaging techniques are continuously improving, providing neuro-ophthalmologists with increasingly detailed maps of brain activity during visual tasks. This allows for a much more nuanced understanding of how the brain processes visual information and identifies the precise areas affected in various neuro-ophthalmological conditions. These refined techniques aid in differentiating between various conditions that might present with similar symptoms, enabling more accurate diagnoses. Furthermore, advanced fMRI protocols can track subtle changes in brain activity over time, monitoring treatment response and disease progression at a level of detail previously unimaginable. The resulting information is crucial for developing personalized treatment plans and understanding the functional consequences of visual system damage. This will enhance the overall effectiveness and precision of neuro-ophthalmological care.

## 7.2 Research Frontiers

The quest for improved visual outcomes hinges on a deeper understanding of the intricate interplay between the nervous system and the eye. Current research focuses intensely on refining existing diagnostic tools and developing entirely novel approaches to treatment. Gene therapy, a rapidly advancing field, offers immense potential. Early clinical trials are already showing promising results in treating inherited retinal diseases, directly addressing the genetic basis of visual impairment. This targeted approach offers a personalized medicine strategy, moving beyond symptomatic treatment to address the root cause of the disorder. Further research is crucial to refine these techniques and broaden their applicability to a wider range of neuro-ophthalmological conditions. We need to move beyond the laboratory and ensure these advancements translate to clinical practice in a safe and effective manner.

One particularly exciting avenue involves the development of advanced neuroimaging techniques. Functional MRI (fMRI) continues to evolve, offering increasingly detailed insights into brain activity associated with visual processing. This allows researchers to map the neural pathways involved in vision with unprecedented accuracy. Improved spatial and temporal resolution opens doors for the identification of subtle abnormalities undetectable with current methods. This enhanced diagnostic capability enables earlier detection and intervention, crucial in conditions where timely treatment significantly improves prognosis. The integration of fMRI with other advanced imaging modalities, such as diffusion tensor imaging (DTI), provides even more comprehensive information on the structural integrity of the visual pathways and the nature of any damage. The potential for earlier and more accurate diagnosis cannot be overstated.

Beyond improved imaging, researchers are actively exploring novel therapeutic strategies. For instance, the development of neuroprotective agents is a high priority. These agents aim to limit the damage caused by various neurological insults to the visual system, such as those occurring in optic neuritis or ischemic optic neuropathy. Preclinical studies using animal models have shown promising results. Identifying effective neuroprotective agents and moving them towards clinical trials is a major focus. This will necessitate rigorous testing to establish efficacy and safety. Careful consideration of the potential side effects and the development of targeted delivery systems will be crucial for success. The ultimate goal is to improve patient outcomes by limiting or preventing visual loss.

Another significant area of focus lies in the realm of stem cell therapy. Studies are investigating the potential of stem cells to regenerate damaged retinal cells or nerve fibers. The ability to replace lost or damaged cells is highly promising. This regenerative approach is being explored in various conditions causing vision loss, including age-related macular degeneration and glaucoma. While still in its early stages, the potential to reverse vision loss due to irreparable cell damage is truly revolutionary. The challenges lie in optimizing the delivery of stem cells, mitigating the risks of rejection, and ensuring long-term survival and integration of the transplanted cells. The meticulous study required highlights this line of research as a long-term project with potentially enormous payoff.

Finally, the integration of artificial intelligence (AI) and machine learning (ML) algorithms into neuro-ophthalmological research is transforming the field. AI can analyze large datasets of imaging data and clinical information, identifying patterns and correlations that might be missed by the human eye. These tools can aid in diagnostics, by improving the accuracy and speed of diagnosis and in treatment planning, by tailoring interventions to the specific needs of individual patients. AI's role in expediting the research process itself cannot be overlooked. AI can optimize experimental design, assist in analyzing complex datasets, and accelerate the development of new therapeutic approaches. Therefore, the careful implementation of these tools represents a crucial aspect of future success. The potential of AI is immense.

www.ingramcontent.com/pod-product-compliance
Lightning Source LLC
LaVergne TN
LVHW022027200926
848481LV00007B/2578
* 9 7 9 8 3 4 9 4 2 4 9 8 4 *